DUNAMIS 2

Living the Resurrected Life

Inner Healing Workbook - Series 2

TIM SOWERS
KEISHA SOWERS

Copyright © 2019 The Sowers Ministries

All rights reserved. No part of this publication may be reproduced, stored in a retrieval system, or transmitted in any form or by any means - for example, electronic, photocopy, recording - without the prior written permission of the authors. The only exception is brief quotations in printed reviews.

ISBN: 978-0-578-59724-9

Interior Design by Machu

Book Cover Design by Machu

Edited by Uzo Nwiyi

Scripture is taken from BibleGateway.com

Some scripture is taken from New International Version.

The Disciple's Study Bible, New International Version ®, NIV®

Copyright © 1988 by Holman Bible Publishers

All rights reserved.

International Copyright secured.

Contents

WHAT IS DUNAMIS 2? 4
HOW TO USE THIS WORKBOOK 5
1 TUNING EMOTIONS 6
2 HOW TO STOP REAPING NEGATIVE HARVESTS 10
3 THE EAGLE 13
4 REMOVING IDOLS 17
5 FEASTING AT THE TABLE 20
6 MINISTERING TO YOURSELF 23
7 OUR VALUE 25
APPENDIX 27
    A. Removing The Enemy's Weapons 28
    B. The KEY OF GRACE 30
    C. The EXCHANGE 31
    D. Building A Case 32
    E. 21 Days Of Gratitude 38
    F. Judgments And Vows 44
CLOSING PRAYER 45
BOOKS AND RESOURCES 46
ABOUT THE AUTHORS 47

What's DUNAMIS 2?

If *dunamis* means "power" in the Greek language, then DUNAMIS 2 is a double portion of that power.

The second workbook in this series focuses on the next level of healing.

DUNAMIS 2 will teach you how to sustain the healing. At the end of this workbook and training, our hope is that you are able to go from glory to glory, and from strength to strength. You may also have the opportunity to help others walk into their healing as well.

Jesus says we will do greater works, and He longs for a relationship with us. He longs for people to know Him, and experience both His crucifixion AND resurrection power in our lives.

Get ready for your double portion!

How To Use This Workbook

We have written this interactive workbook to support you in your healing process. We are praying you finish this journey strong and full of peace. We are also praying that you will help others experience healing through the power of Yeshua so this will cause a ripple effect across the world.

This workbook is not completely self-guiding, but rather a supplement and reference for our sessions and workshops. Inner - healing is best conducted within a safe community. We recommend you schedule a phone, skype, or in-person session with us for the best results.

Keep your heart with all vigilance, for from it flows the springs of life.
Proverbs 4:23

1 TUNING EMOTIONS

When Tim used to work as an engineer, he found himself getting angry while working on field breakdowns or projects.

Coffee Chat With Tim

People would come out while I was working on a job -for example, a production line would be down - so the bosses in that area would keep coming over and asking me,

"Well, when is it going to be done?"

I would say, "I don't know. We're getting there. It's going to take a while before we get there."

A little while later, someone else would come over, someone underneath that manager would come and ask the same question.

I blew it.

I started getting angry and raising my voice, saying tensely, "You're going to have to give me some time to think on this."

The electricians would start laughing because they could see I was getting hot!

Sometimes there would be drawings for the issue and sometimes there wouldn't be. It just took time to figure out how the electrical control was wired up, especially for the older production lines. So, my thought process would be interrupted by all the other questions.

So, I had to learn to control myself when they would come and ask me that question and not respond the way that I had.

I had to ask myself, "What was making me so angry when they would come and ask me those questions?"

I would lose my train of thought due to the questions and would have to go back and regroup and ask the guys I was working with to help me remember where we were in the trouble - shooting process.

Afterwards, I would go and pray and Jesus would say,

"Trust Me to bring back what we've covered before. Your managers needed to get answers for others that needed to know."

After prayer, the Lord would have me go back and apologize to the people who I showed my anger to.

I knew the Lord knew about engineering. He knows all things.

I began to ask the Holy Spirit to go before me and prepare the way to tackle any issues that came up. He would show me things that I didn't know how to do. He would actually at times go before me and by the time I got to the line that was having issues, someone would meet me on the way and let me know that they got it fixed. Amazing!

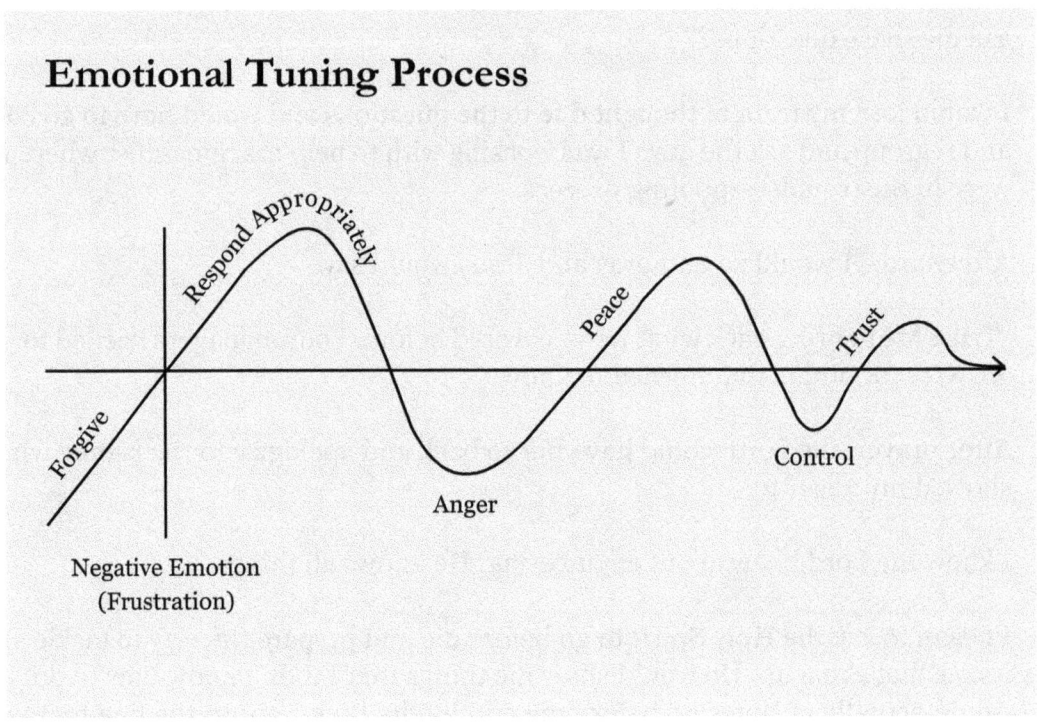

The Tuning Process

So the Holy Spirit gave me an analogy of spiritual progress on, for example, the anger issue, which was, in reality, a fear of getting in trouble for not getting the production line up and running as quick as possible.

At work, we would tune a loop, as it was called, in order to get a process control to the desired setpoint. The Holy Spirit said that in healing there may be several things that needed to be worked on, like tuning a loop.

In tuning a loop, there were several control parameters that needed to be adjusted in order to get the process to maintain a steady control at the desired setpoint.

There were usually 3 tuning parameters: proportional, integral, and derivative. My tuning parameters for this fear were anger, control, and manipulation.

I began to work on the anger part but soon learned that there was more to this as I was tested again in this area.

The next parameter was control. I was trying to control the environment and get what I needed to do as soon as possible. However, the Lord indicated that I shouldn't use that either. After dealing with that, I felt better, however, I still noticed some disturbance inside.

The next thing I had to work on was manipulation. After I worked on that, the spiritual process seemed to be tuned much better and I could respond calmly when folks came out to ask questions.

Of course, I had to forgive and release those folks that I felt were interrupting my process of tuning of trying to help them out. But actually, they were helping me in a more important soul issue.

God does work in mysterious ways, doesn't He?

It is important to keep examining ourselves until we get the whole healing that we are trying to get each time. I wanted to get it over with quickly, but God showed me there were some other inner parameters that needed tuning.

QUESTION:

1. Using the Emotional Tuning Process diagram, write down a negative emotion that you are overcoming. Ask God what are the positive adjustments needed to maintain emotional stability in that area.

Do not be deceived: God cannot be mocked. A man reaps what he sows. Whoever sows to please their flesh, from the flesh will reap destruction; whoever sows to please the Spirit, from the Spirit will reap eternal life. Let us not become weary in doing good, for at the proper time we will reap a harvest if we do not give up.

Galatians 6:7-9

2 HOW TO STOP REAPING NEGATIVE HARVESTS

Do you ever have a dream and sense that it was spiritual?

Dreams are a way that our subconscious speaks to us.

Dreams reveal what is hidden or stuffed down inside of us. Spiritual dreams are one of the ways that God says we are ready to deal with a person or circumstance.

One time, I had a dream that was very disturbing.

In the dream, there were people in my past that had hurt me, people that represented the behaviors of these people of my past, and circumstances where I felt bullied, judged, or dishonored.

Although I say a daily prayer forgiving people and asking for forgiveness, I knew by the depth and intensity of this dream that my subconscious was showing me hidden areas that needed healing.

When I woke up from the dream, I asked God what He wanted me to do about this dream. On several occasions, in answer to my prayer, the Lord instructed me to go back into the dream and physically do and/or say something.

Here is an example of how He instructed me to deal with a dream.

1. Go back to the circumstance in my life where these sorts of events started happening.

2. Ask for forgiveness for my part in that original scene.

3. Pull up the negative seeds of judgment and accusation that I continued to sow towards other people and command the harvest from those seeds to stop growing.

4. Loose angels to go and minister to every person that I hurt, knowingly or unknowingly. Ask God to soften their hearts towards me and forgive me.

5. To remove my name from their thoughts or mouths that was attached to negativity in any way.

6. To ask God to prevent them from ever saying anything negative about me again.

7. To wash me and those involved and the circumstances clean with the blood of Yeshua.

8. To release the dunamis of Yeshua over me, these people, and these circumstances to redeem us and use those situations for good and for God's glory.

After completing the steps, I felt peace. The negative expectations I had of people, which resulted in me being negative, were removed.

Remember, we can only harvest what we have sown and what we expect. If we sow mercy and grace over people, we will receive the same.

QUESTION:

1. What are the ways through which God speaks to you? _____
   _____
   _____
   _____
   _____
   _____
   _____

2. Have you ever had a spiritual dream? If so, what was it about? _____
   _____
   _____
   _____
   _____
   _____
   _____

3. Were you able to deal with your dream and obtain victory or would you like assistance?

4. Ask God to reveal to you any hidden areas in your life where He wants to heal you. Write down those areas here.

5. Schedule a session with us, if possible, if you need support in your healing in the areas listed in #4.

*Those who hope in the Lord will renew their strength.
They will soar on wings like eagles; they will run and not grow weary,
they will walk and not be faint.*
Isaiah 40:31

3 THE EAGLE

One day, while spending time with God, I was praying about some challenges with certain people that were in my life.

We all know in scripture that we are to love our enemies, to pray for them, and even look for opportunities to feed them.

I don't want people to be in pain. I pray for their healing, their salvation, and their deliverance.

However, there are times when the spiritual battle gets weary. Yes, we are called to love people but hate sin. However, sometimes the lines are blurred between the person and the pain that is causing them to treat others with dishonor.

Jesus, while on the cross, had to pass this test and forgive, stating, "they knew not what they were doing".

So, during my prayer time, I saw the vision of a large eagle being given to me.

I was told to climb on top of it whenever I was in an intense situation of warfare. There is a point in altitude God has designed where snakes perish. This is called the "snake line." We know that eagles have the capability of flying above the snake line.

I found it interesting that God would give this spiritual eagle to help in a time of need. There are supporting scriptures that explain this vision better.

In Exodus 19:4, "You yourselves have seen what I have did to Egypt, and how I carried you on eagles' wings and brought you to myself."

In Isaiah 40:31, "But those who hope in the Lord will renew their strength. They will soar on wings like eagles; they will run and not grow weary, they will walk and not be faint."

Revelations 12:14, The woman was given the two wings of a great eagle, so that she might fly to the place prepared for her in the wilderness, where she would be taken care of for a time, times and half a time, out of the serpent's reach."

CHALLENGE:

In addition to the spiritual eagle, how can we take a practical approach to "level up" in life?

What happens if we change our perspective about "difficult people?"

What if we look at ourselves instead and see how challenging people can actually be beneficial to our own growth?

_____
_____
_____
_____
_____
_____
_____
_____
_____
_____
_____
_____
_____
_____
_____
_____
_____
_____
_____

Collaboration Exercise

1. **See difficult people as teachers.** They may be in your life to teach you a valuable lesson.

What can you learn from a difficult person in your life? What lessons can you pick up from interacting with this person? Even if it's only to teach you patience, they are valuable to you in some way.

_____
_____
_____
_____
_____
_____
_____
_____
_____

Why does this person remain in your life?

_____
_____
_____
_____
_____
_____
_____
_____
_____

2. **See difficult people as messengers.** Perhaps they're revealing to you a part of your personality that could use some work or healing. They may trigger thoughts and feelings in you that require some thought and soul searching.

For example, a person who annoys you with constant talking may be triggering the part of you that could work on communication. Why are you bothered by the extensive talking, and what does it really mean?

_____
_____
_____
_____
_____
_____
_____
_____
_____

3. **Learn to change reactions.** If a difficult person cannot be avoided, it will benefit you to learn to live with them. **One method to embrace this type of person involves learning to change your reaction.** How can you change your reaction to this person next time?

_____
_____
_____
_____
_____
_____
_____
_____
_____

You may be used to reacting to this person with anger or frustration. However, if you reacted with calmness and understanding instead, **not only will it put you in control of the interaction, but you might also discover a whole new facet of their personality.**

It is important to keep in mind that even difficult people have feelings and can get hurt. **They need love and understanding just as much or more than anyone else.** Change your reaction to them and you might even find a new friend.

Dr. Nicolya Williams **(credit:** https://www.nicolyawilliams.com/**)** and Certified Coaches Alliance (CCA) (https://certifiedcoachesalliance.com/) developed an effective strategy to increase our capacity to collaborate.

> *For God so loved the world, that He gave His only begotten Son, that whosoever believeth in Him should not perish, but have everlasting life.*
> John 3:16

4 REMOVING IDOLS

Prophetic word given during prayer time, October 4, 2019

If you cannot hear from Me at times, consider the blockage.

What is occupying your soul and heart?

What is taking up the most room?

Where is your time devoted throughout the day?

Relationship with Me should be priority in all you do
Even in your work

The longer you spend with Me
The more you will know the truth
And the more you will know the truth about yourself...
Why and how I designed you.

Remove the blockages and the mute idols and the lies
Then you can clearly hear from Me
And get to know your Creator –
The one who truly loves you.

I AM the One who loves you and longs for you.
I AM devoted to you and pursue your heart and want the best for you.
I know you better than you know yourself.

So many go to self-help, but
I AM the one who knows you and can help you
If you let Me.

Action:

1. Do you currently have idols? Pray and see what Holy Spirit reveals to you.

2. Meditate on Hebrews 8:9-13. Take notes and ask Holy Spirit for revelation on this scripture as it pertains to your life.

3. Meditate on Hebrews 4:12-16. Write down what is revealed to you.

4. Craft your own heart response or prayer of dedication to God.

You prepare a table before me in the presence of my enemies. You anoint my head with oil; my cup overflows.

Psalm 23:5

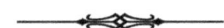

5 FEASTING AT THE TABLE

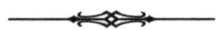

In Dunamis 1, Chapter 5, we discussed the power of Fasting. Now, in Dunamis 2, we will share the revelation of Feasting in both traditional and symbolic context.

Symbolic Occasion For Feasting

What does Psalm 23, verse 5 say? It says He prepares a table before us in the presence of our enemies. He anoints our head with oil, and our cup runs over.

Our enemies are not going to be in heaven. That means, God is preparing a table for us now in the physical realm. Why are we waiting to get to heaven to partake of what God is giving us now? Why are we waiting to get to heaven to feast at the table?

We eat when we are hungry, we don't eat when we're full. So we must get rid of shame, offense, bitterness, unforgiveness, sorrow and other hindrances so we can feast at the table. We must let go of them from within as we exchange them for God's goodness.

Let us eat and feast from the table Our Father has prepared for us.

Take a moment and do the exchange.

Please go to Appendix C for guidance on how to do this.

Traditional Occasions For Feasting

Although some believe there is no longer a need to observe the Holy Days because they were part of Old Testament tradition, note that Jesus also observed them in the New Testament.

As Tim and I have grown in our walk with Yeshua, we have felt a desire to observe the Holy Days. We have become closer to our Jewish friends because of this, and we enjoy travelling to Israel to research and learn more about Jewish culture.

Leviticus 23 outlines the types of traditional feasting days to be observed.

Here is a brief overview.

The Spring Feasts
    Passover
    Unleavened Bread
    First Fruits
    Pentecost

The Fall Feasts
    Trumpets
    Atonement
    Tabernacles

Weekly Feast - The Sabbath

Action:
1. Research in the Bible where these feasts occurred. Write down the scriptures below. (Hint: Leviticus 23 is a great start)

___
___
___
___
___
___
___
___
___
___
___

2. Why did these feasts take place?

3. What was eaten and is there symbolism in the food?

4. Write your own revelation about the importance of feasting with God and His people.

> *"Physician, heal thyself."*
> Luke 4:23

6 MINISTERING TO YOURSELF

I am fully convinced that God allows us to go through trials and tribulations so He can carry us through them. We will then have a testimony to help others through similar situations.

Case in point, after years and years of reading books and ministering to others on emotional wellness, I am constantly challenged in this area. No matter the tools we have taught, the people we have trained, there are times when I have to call on my husband to help me work through an issue I'm having. We are usually rewarded with additional revelation on the inner - healing process.

Recently, Tim walked me through one of these moments and stopped. He said, "If you were to minister to yourself right now, what would you say to yourself?"

Hmmm.

It reminded me of Luke 4:23, when Jesus spoke to the Nazarenes, "Surely you will quote this proverb to me: 'Physician, heal yourself!'"

You see, with the Holy Spirit being our Counselor, we have the answers we need already inside of us.

Living an empowered life is working with Holy Spirit to find the answers and being wise enough to use the tools that He has given us.

CHALLENGE:
1. Is there an area in your life that you are constantly overcoming?

___

2. Incorporating the tools from *Dunamis 1* and *Dunamis 2*, if you were to minister to yourself, what would you say or do to get a breakthrough?

For you created my inmost being; you knit me together in my mother's womb. 14 I praise you because I am fearfully and wonderfully made; your works are wonderful, I know that full well. 15 My frame was not hidden from you when I was made in the secret place, when I was woven together in the depths of the earth. 16 Your eyes saw my unformed body; all the days ordained for me were written in your book before one of them came to be. 17 How precious to me are your thoughts, God! How vast is the sum of them! 18 Were I to count them, they would outnumber the grains of sand— when I awake, I am still with you.

Psalm 139:13-18

7 OUR VALUE

God loves us so much. Even when it is time to pass on, He still pursues us and longs for us to choose Him for eternity. This is how much He values us.

In this chapter, we are sharing the story of Sam Tinsley, who was instructed by God to share the love of Jesus with a woman who stopped breathing in the hospital.

This story is told by his former wife, Cheryl. (Sam has passed, gone home to be with God.)

Going after the one
As told by Cheryl Tinsley Hood

Yes, the story Sam often told at CARE group and shared as part of his testimony was incredible. I too miss his stories and the blessing that he was to all of us.

This particular story was about a family member of a parishioner who was in ICU. The patient was not a believer so the parishioner asked Sam if he would go visit her in the hospital to share the gospel of Jesus with her.

When he arrived, the ICU nurse said that he was too late. She had passed away moments earlier. Sam was going to leave but the Holy Spirit prompted him to go into her room anyway. He wrestled momentarily with God over this, but God clearly told him to go in and speak to her, so he did.

He told her that Jesus loved her and died on a cross for all of us so that we could live eternally with him. He prayed over her and then told her that if she could hear Him, all she had to do was confess her sin and ask Jesus to forgive her and be the Lord of her life.

As he continued to pray, what had been a steady flat line on her cardiac monitor began to bleep. Her family was in the room with Sam and witnessed this, which they all believe was the moment at which she received Jesus as Lord and Savior.

Sam gave this testimony to encourage all who hear or sense God's calling to be obedient even when circumstances seem as though they are impossible. God can do the impossible through us when we trust Him and are obedient.

1. The dunamis of Yeshua brings life. What is He saying to you right now? Do you sense God is calling you to share His love in a current situation?

2. This story is a testament of how valuable we all are to Him. How has this affected your own sense of purpose?

APPENDIX

APPENDIX A

REMOVING THE ENEMY'S WEAPONS

Wounds in our bodies can sometimes be from enemy attacks when we open the door.

1 Peter 5:8 Peter tells us to stay alert and watch out for your great enemy, the devil. He prowls around like a roaring lion, looking for someone to devour.

2 Corinthians 10:5 We demolish arguments and every pretension that sets itself up against the knowledge of God, and we take captive every thought to make it obedient to Christ.

Ephesians 6:10 A final word: Be strong in the Lord and in his mighty power. 11 Put on all of God's armor so that you will be able to stand firm against all strategies of the devil. 12 For we are not fighting against flesh-and-blood enemies, but against evil rulers and authorities of the unseen world, against mighty powers in this dark world, and against evil spirits in the heavenly places. 13 Therefore, put on every piece of God's armor so you will be able to resist the enemy in the time of evil. Then after the battle you will still be standing firm. 14 Stand your ground, putting on the belt of truth and the body armor of God's righteousness. 15 For shoes, put on the peace that comes from the Good News so that you will be fully prepared. 16 In addition to all of these, hold up the shield of faith to stop the fiery arrows of the devil. 17 Put on salvation as your helmet, and take the sword of the Spirit, which is the word of God.
18 Pray in the Spirit at all times and on every occasion. Stay alert and be persistent in your prayers for all believers everywhere.

As we read these scriptures, we realize that we are in a spiritual battle and as a result we may get wounded. This could occur when we dwell on negative thoughts so much or as a result of someone saying negative things about us or when someone has said something that hurts us.

I have found in the past that spiritual weapons can become stuck in us.

For instance, arrows, darts, swords and spears have had to be removed from persons I have prayed for and within myself. I usually see these in the spiritual realm as the Holy Spirit points them out.

Steps To Remove Spiritual Weapons From The Enemy

1. *Prayer*
   I usually pray like this, "Father, I plead the blood of Jesus over myself and the person being prayed for and any other people present. I ask for Your protection and guidance in this prayer as I reach in the spirit realm and pull this arrow out of the person."
2. *Destroy it*
   As I pull it out, I then ask an angel to come and take it to destroy it or I cast it away and command it to dematerialize.
3. *Healing of the Wound*
   I then ask Holy Spirit to remove any poison that may have been left inside and to bring healing from the inside out.
4. *New Armor*
   I then ask for a new piece of armor to cover the area that was wounded.

APPENDIX B
THE KEY OF GRACE

The years of preparation before marriage, God would give me items in the spirit realm. One day, He handed me a key. I inquired what it was.

He said, "This is the Key of Grace. This is the key that will give you access to your husband's heart."

He then shared there are so many people praying for a spouse, but they are hindering the process because of judgment and criticism when they meet a potential person.

He showed me that peoples' hearts are full of treasure, and in order to access their hearts, there must be a key, just like there is a key to a chest.

If you have been wounded by people in the past, there is healing available to you. You do not have to walk around bitter, cynical, jaded, or full of fear. You are encouraged to do the Exchange in Appendix C.

So many people are bound with the fear of rejection or of being hurt.

However, perfect love casts out all fear. Perfect, unconditional love can only be found in Our Heavenly Father.

The essence of marriage is perfecting love, not finding perfect love.

Ask Father God for the Key of Grace for people, as you rest in His perfect love.

APPENDIX C
THE EXCHANGE

There are spiritual exchanges that take place in Isaiah 61.

As you enter into the Secret Place with the
Most High during your prayer time you
can do the exchange shown in verse 3.

You do not have to keep ashes, for He'll bestow
on you a crown of beauty.
Instead of mourning, He will give you oil of gladness.
Instead of a spirit of despair, we can put on a garment of praise.

I encourage you to spend intimate time with The Most High daily
and see the exchanges from negative to positive outcomes take place in your life.

"Instead of their shame my people will receive a double portion,
and instead of disgrace they will rejoice in their inheritance;
and so they will inherit a double portion in their land,
and everlasting joy will be theirs." Isaiah 61: 7

APPENDIX D
BUILDING A CASE

One of the ways the enemy tries to destroy us is through our identity as children of God. He will try to insert doubt, division, or distraction in a situation to influence you to see people or circumstances from a negative perspective.

He is the accuser of the brethren, so he will try to prevent you from fulfilling your purpose and life assignments. Jesus said the greatest commandments are to "love God and love people." If we don't trust God or people, the enemy has succeeded in preventing us from tapping into *dunamis.*

To counter this, we can look at scripture to see how Adam handled it in Genesis and then in the New Testament to observe Jesus sharing the correct way.

When the enemy tries to build a case and insert doubt, Jesus would choose to see people or situations the way His Father does.

When the enemy tried to speak through others to cause anxiety and lack, Jesus would posture Himself with gratitude and trust that God would protect and provide.

When the enemy would work through others to distract and discourage Yeshua, Jesus forgave and continued to focus on completing His assignments for God.

Activation:

1. Using the chart on the next page, we want you to list areas in your life where the enemy has skewed your perspective.
2. In the middle column, write down what God is doing in this situation.
3. In the third column, record any scriptures Holy Spirit gives you regarding this situation and decree them over your life.
4. In the fourth column, write down your testimony. These are milestones to build a case against the enemy the next time he tries to insert doubt, division, or distraction.

The Accuser	What Is God Doing?	Scripture Meditation & Decree	Testimony
1			
2			
3			
4			
5			

The Accuser	What Is God Doing?	Scripture Meditation & Decree	Testimony
1			
2			
3			
4			
5			

The Accuser	What Is God Doing?	Scripture Meditation & Decree	Testimony
1			
2			
3			
4			
5			

21 DAYS OF GRATITUDE

Changing your perspective to give thanks in all things, in all circumstances, will empower you for abundance. Over the next 21 days, list 5 things you are grateful for and any particular highlights of that day in the Notes section. This assignment will help recalibrate your lifestyle, positioning you for healing and breakthrough.

DAY 1

1. _____
2. _____
3. _____
4. _____
5. _____

NOTES

DAY 2

1. _____
2. _____
3. _____
4. _____
5. _____

DAY 3

1. _____
2. _____
3. _____
4. _____
5. _____

21 DAYS OF GRATITUDE

DAY 4

1. _____
2. _____
3. _____
4. _____
5. _____

DAY 5

1. _____
2. _____
3. _____
4. _____
5. _____

DAY 6

1. _____
2. _____
3. _____
4. _____
5. _____

DAY 7

1. _____
2. _____
3. _____
4. _____
5. _____

NOTES

21 DAYS OF GRATITUDE

DAY 8

1. _____
2. _____
3. _____
4. _____
5. _____

NOTES

DAY 9

1. _____
2. _____
3. _____
4. _____
5. _____

DAY 10

1. _____
2. _____
3. _____
4. _____
5. _____

DAY 11

1. _____
2. _____
3. _____
4. _____
5. _____

21 DAYS OF GRATITUDE

DAY 12

1. _____
2. _____
3. _____
4. _____
5. _____

NOTES

DAY 13

1. _____
2. _____
3. _____
4. _____
5. _____

DAY 14

1. _____
2. _____
3. _____
4. _____
5. _____

DAY 15

1. _____
2. _____
3. _____
4. _____
5. _____

21 DAYS OF GRATITUDE

DAY 16

1. _____
2. _____
3. _____
4. _____
5. _____

NOTES

DAY 17

1. _____
2. _____
3. _____
4. _____
5. _____

DAY 18

1. _____
2. _____
3. _____
4. _____
5. _____

DAY 19

1. _____
2. _____
3. _____
4. _____
5. _____

21 DAYS OF GRATITUDE

DAY 20

1. _____
2. _____
3. _____
4. _____
5. _____

DAY 21

1. _____
2. _____
3. _____
4. _____
5. _____

NOTES

APPENDIX F
JUDGMENTS AND VOWS

In the first DUNAMIS workbook (Chapter 6 - Truth Meditation), Tim revealed he made judgments against his earthly father. He revealed how those judgments were keeping him in bondage and the vows actually caused him to be just like his father.

For DUNAMIS 2, we want to give you the strategy to release your own judgments and vows to break free.

Step 1: Ask the Lord to reveal the judgments and vows made contributing to the heart issue. There are usually three or four (but could be more).

Judgments	**Vow**
1.	
2.	
3.	
4.	
5.	

Step 2: After listing them you may want to pray a prayer similar to this:

"Lord, I confess and repent for my sin of making these judgments and vows and for coming into agreement with them. Forgive me for believing these lies. I forgive the person or institution for any way they have wounded me and release them, they owe me nothing. And I bless them in every way. I also forgive myself. I break the power of these judgments and vows over me and declare them null and void. They will no longer affect me in any way. Please stop the reaping of what I have sown. In the name of your son, Yeshua, I pray. Amen."

CLOSING PRAYER

Father God,

We thank you for leading this brave soul into your resurrection power.

We pray for wisdom and strength over them to use these tools and for hope to rise up within them.

We thank you for the healing that has already taken place and pray that the Holy Spirit will continue to regenerate them into how you have designed them.

We cancel out any retribution or backlash from the enemy. We ask for your angels to protect our readers and envelop them with your love and power.

May they go from glory to glory, strength to strength!

We pray this in the name of your son, Yeshua, the one who died and rose again for us.

Amen.

BOOKS AND RESOURCES

Dr. Henry W. Wright, *A More Excellent Way* (Whitaker House, includes DVD edition, 2009), 544 pages

Tim and Keisha Sowers, *DUNAMIS: Living the Resurrected Life* (Florida: The Sowers Ministries, 2019), 53 pages

Mark and Patti Virkler, *Prayers that Heal the Heart* (Bridge-Logos Publishers, 2001), 320 pages

Roderick C. Meredith, *The Holy Days: God's Master Plan* (Living Church of God, 2017), 47 pages

ABOUT THE AUTHORS

Tim and Keisha Sowers are the founders of The Sowers Ministries.

They have written several books and host healing retreats and training in West Palm Beach, Florida USA to empower people in the inner healing process. They would love to hear from you and support you on your spiritual journey.

Instagram @thesowersfamily
Facebook TimandKeisha Sowers

www.ingramcontent.com/pod-product-compliance
Lightning Source LLC
Chambersburg PA
CBHW080443170426
43195CB00017B/2872